First Aid for First Responders

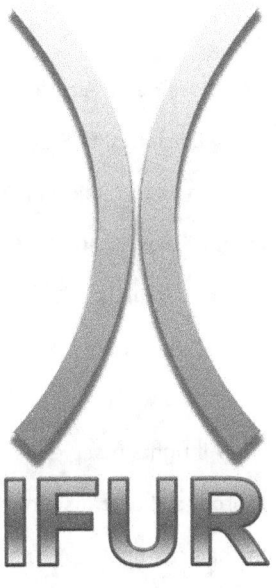

IFUR

Investigación y Formación
en Urgencias

1

© 2015 José Pérez Vigueras, Jose Perez Alcaraz, Ana Laura Barrera Vallejo

© Ediciones IFUR SL

Edited by Research and Training in Emergency SL

C / Workers Tana 17, 30570, Beniaján

Murcia

Ifur@ifur.es

Www.ifur.es

ISBN-13: 978-1540407979

ISBN-10: 1540407977

Printed in Charleston - USA

FIRST EDITION

THANKS

The authors wish to thank our friends and family by It received support in developing this project. Y, Above all, to thank Research and Training in Emergency SL His unconditional trust without which it would have been impossible develop this project. Thanks to all that you have made it possible to develop this guide First Aid for the whole family.

PROLOGUE

It is difficult to start prefacing a book that you've Dedicated many hours of work and sum it up in just A few words. It 's been almost ten years since We published our first book and continue with the same Idea to show our knowledge and get better Life for those who care about her and the Loved ones around them . This small guide wants and claims to be from his humble Modesty a simple way but very useful and practical in those Times when the same nerves prevent us act And we not know what to do; in it, the reader will find advice Based on the experience of many professionals who It will solve any doubt a pleasant and direct. Finally, say that is a real pride to see grow a Idea and see it reflected in this book. One idea that as All restless people tormenting us to see it done Reality.

José Pérez Vigueras

INTRODUCTION

First aid is urgent measures apply to victims of accidents or sudden illnesses to have specialized medical care. Its purpose is none other than relieve pain and anxiety of the injured/sick and prevent aggravates the state in which it is located. Usually they vary according to the needs of the victim and according to knowledge rescuer. knowing what not to do is as important as knowing what to do. emergency situations are characterized by the need for quick solutions and the time effective.

The purpose of this guide is to provide effective solutions to anyone who at some point are faced with a emergency.

In this guide we address different situations related to characteristics from performance before emergency, yes as basic cardiopulmonary resuscitation (CPR) techniques first aid, how to deal with bleeding, fractures, burns, fainting, intoxication, etc., learning to recognize the signs and related symptoms. Above all basic health education.

INDEX OF AUTHORS

José Pérez Vigueras Expert in Emergency and Catastrophe. Emergency Management

Ana Laura Barrera Vallejo Emergency nurse and Hospitalization

José Pérez Alcaraz Health Emergency Technician.

INDEX

1. EMERGENCY SYSTEMS. ACTIVATION SYSTEM. FAMILY INFORMATION. MEANS AVAILABLE

Currently, all emergency systems are Concentrated on a single phone number 911, who Responsible for filtering calls and organize emergency as Required, either medical equipment, fire, police, etc.

We must teach anyone to use this number When they witness an emergency and they are alone. We will emphasize 9-1-1 numbers separately, as it is easier Remembered by children and the elderly. We never refer to it as A figure, "nine hundred elven".

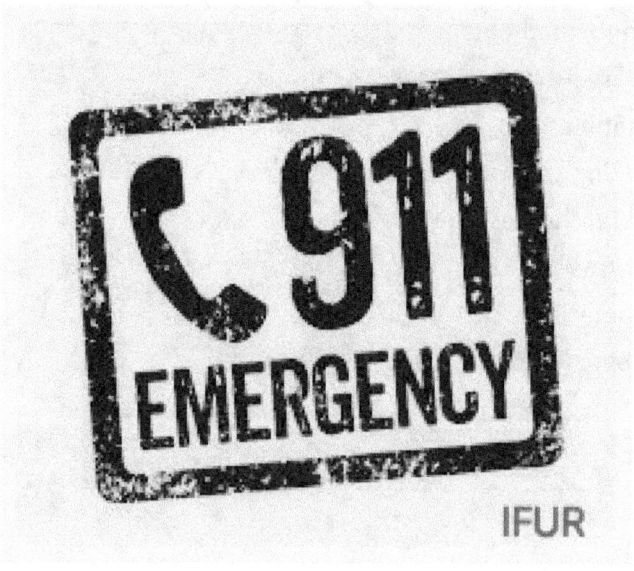

IFUR

Whenever an emergency or emergency arises, We must activate the emergency chain putting us in touch Using said phone number to receive assistance As soon as possible. If the emergency occurs within the center Educational communication of what happened to the family is required A priority.

What to do:

- Keep calm
- Protect yourself and the injured, 911 and ask for help Succor to the injured person, always in that order
- Prevent further injury occurring
- Check that the scene where the victim is safe
- Wait for rescue teams, if necessary

What NOT to do:

- Focus our attention to the obvious
- Act if you are not sure or not clear what can do. Do not act unless you know how to do it
- Touching the wound unprotected area
- Move the victim, especially if you have suffered trauma
- Administer medication

Mainly we should remain calm and try to solve the problem of the quickest and most effective way for the injured you feel safer.

2. FIRST AID KIT

It is important to the school or at home a first aid kit to administer first aid effective. First Aid kits can be purchased in boxes marketed, they can be facilitated by labor mutual relevant or manufacture it ourselves accidents. Here we describe the materials must contain such

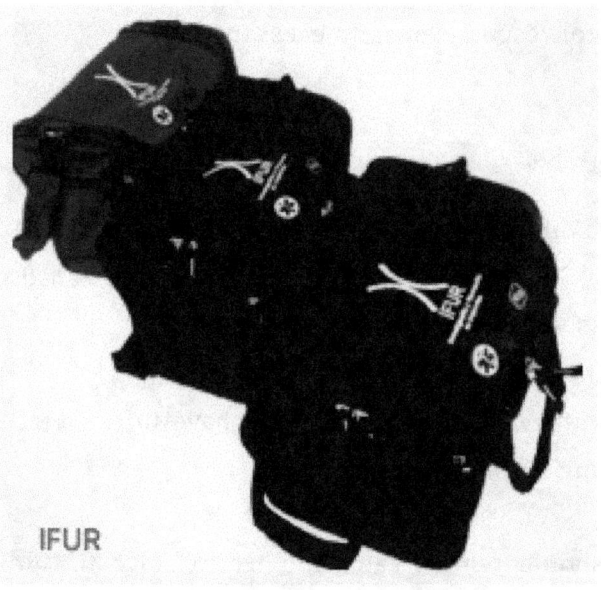

IFUR

The medicine kit bag first aid, should be easy to transport and quickly into reachable

Kit:

- Adhesive bandages, dressings or bandages: available in a wide variety of sizes and for all types of cuts

- Crepe bandages or gauze wound: allow free movement and are recommended to ensure gauzes and / or pads they are what we use for wounds that are difficult us corking

- Gauze dressings: are soft and absorbent pads they provide a good environment to heal wounds and corking bleedings. This is recommended for cleaning wounds, sealing bleeding, burns, etc.

- Plaster: tapes are of various sizes, consisting of water resistant adhesive. We will use it to hold bandages. We will have two types: fabric, especially if they will not be in contact with the skin, and paper, for skins sensitive.

- Other optional elements: digital thermometer, tweezers, scissors, safety pins, antiseptic (never iodized) solution and solution salt, paracetamol and ibuprofen in syrup, and a bag thermal.

3. BASIC TECHNIQUES IN CPR (REANIMATION CARDIOPULMONARY) IN CHILDREN AND ADULTS

Reanimation cardiopulmonary or CPR is the set of maneuvers that identify when a person In cardiac arrest or PCR, and initiate timely maneuvers that will help us replace the functions Respiratory and circulatory, as soon as possible, until Is treated by medical services.

The steps are:

- Check the level of consciousness. We will go to the person asking how find, noting if it moves or makes a noise. In for babies, we hit them gently plant standing, looking to cry.
- Ask for help, if no response is received.
- Open the airway. We will head tilt - chin. Place a hand on the forehead and the index finger and heart of the other hand adjourn the chin, tilting her head Behind. Hand adjourn the chin, tilting her head Behind.

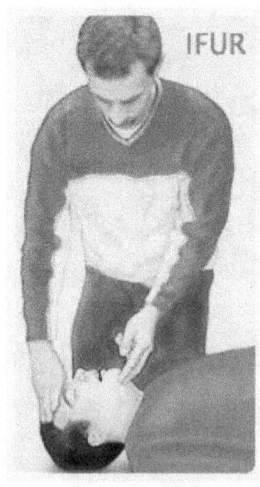

- We will look inside the mouth to confirm that no there is the presence of any foreign body. If possible your withdrawal try it with your fingers, never realizing swept blindly.
- Check breathing. SEE, HEAR and FEEL we place them near our ear nose and mouth victim, looking at the victim's chest and checking breathing for about 10 seconds. If breathing, place a the victim in recovery or PLS position.

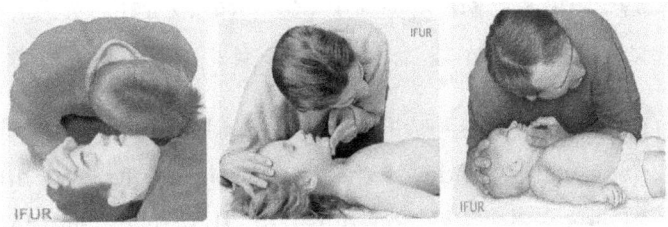

- If not breathing, start artificial respiration. We will stand by the head of the victim opening the airway. We will cover your child's nose with one hand, we place our mouth around the victim's mouth forming an airtight seal and will blow air.

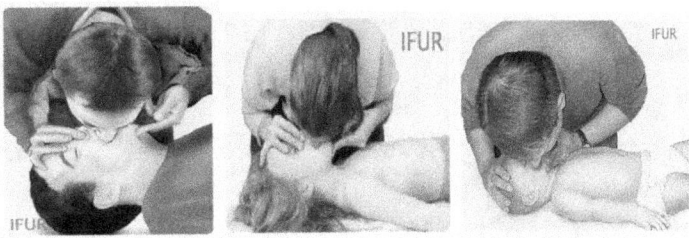

- We will 2 breaths, with an interval of 4 Seconds between the two and maintaining the position of the head.
- The swelling volume will depend on the lung capacity of the victim. For example, if you were a baby insufflation air volume corresponds to the volume of air our oral cavity. If we have a barrier method, such as masks CPR, would be advisable to use as method of protection for those involved.

In the new 2015 AHA recommendations this step is not strictly necessary to do so ; so, if we are not sure do well, we will focus only on the chest compressions.

- Check the pulse. Will place the index and middle fingers on the neck victim aside of the trachea in adults and prepuberant; in babies will check the pulse on the inside of the arm. We will check the pulse for at least 10 seconds. If you have a pulse, continue airing until arrival of aid

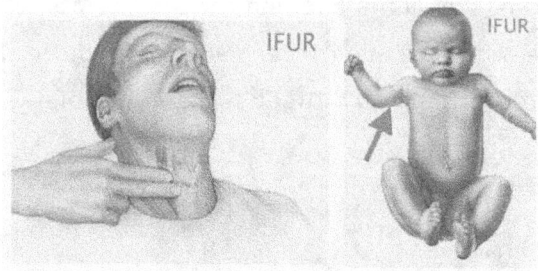

- If no pulse, begin chest compressions. We will place the heel of the hand in the middle of the sternum, to the height of the nipples. We will place the other hand on top, intertwining the fingers of both and apply pressure down compressing a third chest, leaving behind which the chest to return to its initial position. We will do 30 compressions rhythmically to a rate of 120 compressions per minute.

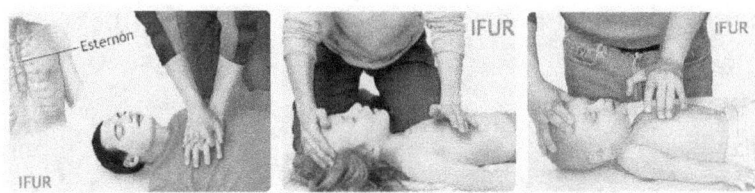

- In infants use 2 fingers for perform the compressions; children use one hand. We will five cycles of 30 compressions and 2 inflations. Reevaluate to the victim each five cycles and we continue CPR until the arrival of services health.

4. POISONING AND POISONING

The most common poisonings occur with products Caustics and corrosives. Be especially careful with Drugs and chemicals in their containers Original.

If a person has taken a toxic substance may present Burns around the mouth and that nauseated usual, Vomits or has diarrhea.

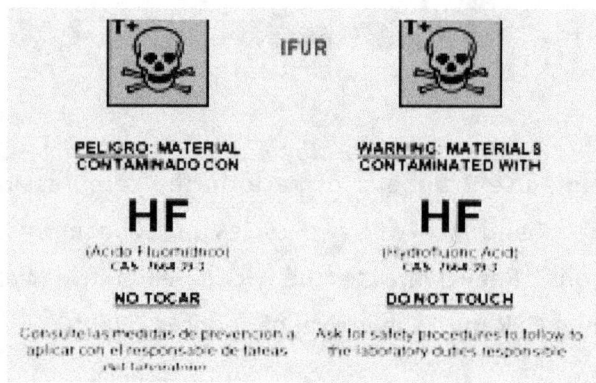

The first thing to do before poisoning is to remove the victim of the toxic product.

- If the product is in solid form, such as tablets, do not perform digital scans blindly and encourage expel or coughing
- If it is a gas, you may need a mask to protect himself . After reviewing the area for safety, remove the the area and take victim to fresh air. Ventilate the area if possible
- If it is corrosive to the skin, remove the clothing and wash the

affected area with plenty of water. Keep the container or label product

- If the toxic product is in contact with the eyes, wash the eyes with plenty of water
- If there is any doubt: Toxicology information service the American Association of Poison Control Centers supports the nation's 55 poison centers in their efforts to prevent and treat poison exposures. Poison centers offer free, confidential medical advice 24 hours a day, seven days a week through the Poison Help line at 1-800-222-1222. This service provides a primary resource for poisoning information and helps reduce costly hospital visits through in-home treatment.

5. ALLERGIES

An allergic reaction is a sensitivity to a specific substance called an allergen, that is contacted through the skin, of the lungs, has been swallowed or injected. The body's reaction can be mild, like a rash localized, or mortal, like anaphylactic shock. The most common allergens include:

- Foods
- Medicines
- Insect bites
- Latex

How to act in case of reactions ranging from mild to moderate
- We must calm the victim, as anxiety can increase the speed of evolution reaction
- You need to identify the allergen and cause them to avoid contact with it in the future
- If you have an itchy rash, should be applied cold compresses. We must avoid using medicated lotions
- If you have at hand a drug emergency cases allergy, will help inject the drug. Avoid administering oral medications if the victim has breathlessness
- Pay attention especially to allergies Intolerance to eggs and cow's milk. Before any symptom is an urgent need to use the services of emergency

How to act in case of severe allergic reactions (anaphylaxis):
- Measures should be taken to prevent shock (falling blood

pressure, preventing blood supply to organs vital important: heart, lung and brain). Will place the victim in a horizontal position, will raise his legs and we will cover it with a coat

- If blacked out , place it on the position lateral safety (PLS) and call 911
- Seek medical attention. We examine the airway, breathing and circulation. A sign will consider and that warns us of sore throat is a voice very hoarse or whispered, or grunting sounds when the victim is Inhaling air. If you have difficulty breathing, weakness extreme or unconsciousness, call immediately emergency medical service and start with the rescue breathing and CPR

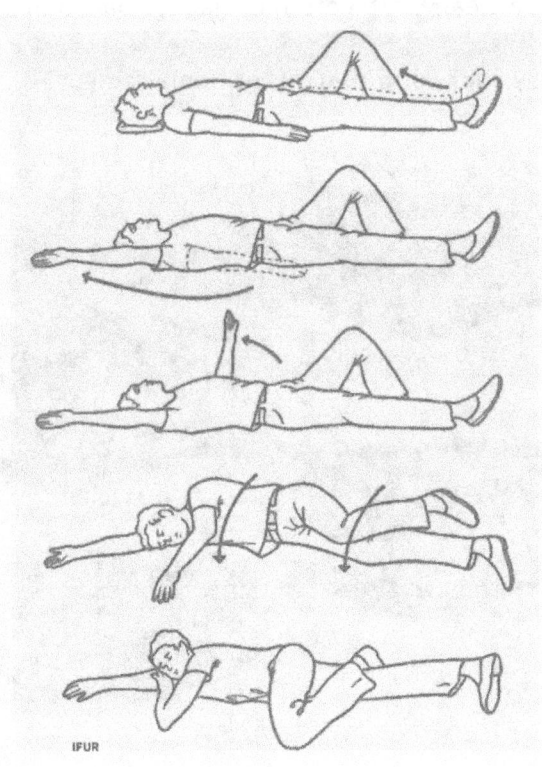

19

6. BURNS

There are different types of burns, but the treatment for one is very similar:

Thermal burns

They are burns caused by fire, hot liquids, friction, etc.

If the burn is small keep it completely under water For a long time or until the discomfort disappears. If the clothing is stuck to the skin, do not try to remove it , just remove it cutting it if it is not attached. Cover the wound with a clean cloth cotton or gauze soaked in sterile saline.

Do not apply any soap, or ointment, or home remedy.

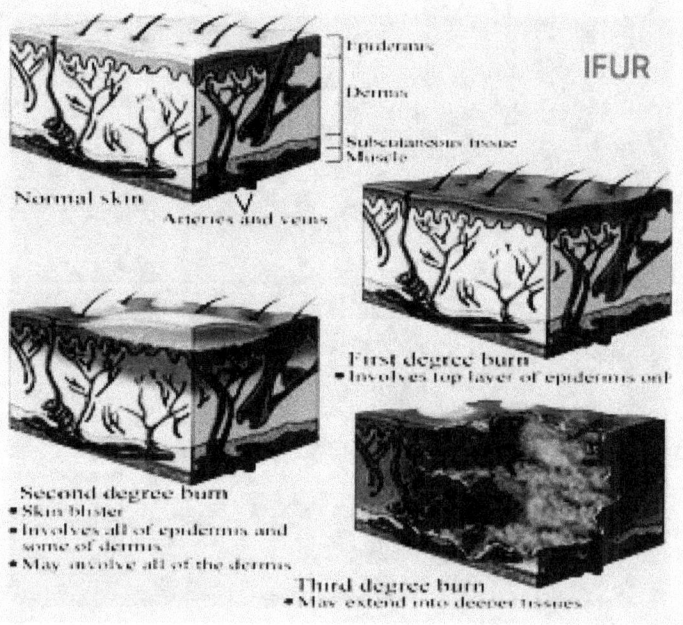

If the burn is extensive, do not offer anything to drink or eat. Ask for help emergency system. Keep the victim covered with a blanket to maintain normal temperature body until medical help arrives.

Electrical burns

It is very important to personal protection, avoiding contact Live with the person while in contact with the current power.

If you are still in contact with the electrical current, electricity will travel through the body of the victim and electrify you too, so we must turn off the power and separate from the power source with an insulating object (wood, plastic, etc.).

Once the victim is free of the current, it is priority check your level of consciousness, airway and review check for a pulse. When the victim is stable, wet with cold water the burns.

Do not move the victim and lay hold on floor.

Do not touch burns, do not use soap, or ointments and any home remedy. After washing the burn, apply clean cotton cloth soaked in saline in Burn.

Whenever there have been electrical burns You activate the emergency system, keeping warm the victim.

7. FALLS AND STROKES

Tips to Avoid Them

- Always try to have good lighting at home
- To access high places using stable stairs; the stools can be dangerous
- Put a non - slip material on the floor of the tub
- For cleaning floors using products that do not become a slippery surface. Avoid stepping on soil wet
- Never leave a young child alone on a surface Elevated
- Place high railings or safety latches on the dangerous places
- The order of the house is helpful to prevent accidents
- It is cautious when making activities involving some Risk
- Be careful with small carpets
- Always use proper footwear and protections if you go to Perform some activity (cycling, skating, ...)

Bruises

It is recommended to apply ice packs or bags so Indirectly in the body part that has suffered the injury immediately after the event and apply it slightly Pressure. The ice pack should be held at least 20 Minutes and can alternate with a heating pad during 48 hours. The hematoma has to go through the stages Appropriate healing before disappearing, changing color Red to purple, to yellow and then brown.

Head injuries

The skull-brain injury (TBI) is one of the accidents more frequent; and according to the magnitude of the coup and symptoms that occur are classified as mild, moderate and severe; depending on this, the required attention is different so As the need to perform studies such as x - rays skull and even tomographic (CT).

It is important to clarify what occurred height fall, symptoms that accompany the event, loss of alertness or fainting, convulsions, vomiting, confusion or irritability, somnolence and abnormal gait. The presence of any of these data must be absolute indication of search timely care.

Warning signs before a blow to the head

- Blackouts
- Asymmetric pupils or anisocoria
- Tendency to fall asleep despite stimulation
- Blurry vision
- Inability to move or feel any part of the body
- Inability to recognize people or places
- Inability to speak or see
- Inability to maintain balance
- Important otic or nosebleed
- Liquid Clear Coming out By Nose Or Mouth (liquid Cerebrospinal)
- Severe headache

Sprains and fractures (fx)

It is necessary to immobilize the limb, resting and applying local cold. If pain or swelling persists, consult a doctor.

Amputations

With sterile gauze wrap the affected part and lobbying In the area in the event of active bleeding. We must do everything possible to preserve the amputated part, keeping it in closed plastic bag and surrounding it with a cloth, applying around ice and water (never with ice directly). In case of partial separation, will be maintained no matter how small the union.

Loss of teeth the tooth

Should be stored in a container with water, solution saline or milk, although not necessary in children up to 3 and 4 years in which these teeth are not definitive.
If the piece is part of permanent teeth, go to a Dentist as soon as possible reimplantation of it.

Before a stroke, seek medical assistance if:

- The injury is due to serious accident
- There are marks of bruises or hematomas important
- Significant hematomas occur with minimal injury
- If severe pain, redness, swelling or presents warmth to touch accompanying

The bruise makeshift detention

When we witness a bump or bruise, while arrive emergency services can immobilize the injured with the materials that we have. Any material we find can serve and help immobilization.

- A long rolled towel at both ends and put Below the neck and neck, you can help to immobilize the area Like a collar. Then you just have to immobilize The head by a tape passing through the front and Chin.

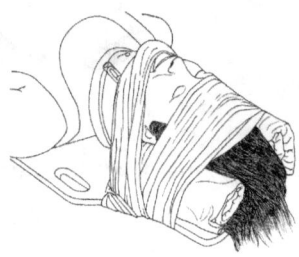

- With a scarf, handkerchief or other cloth to fill A newspaper or magazine folded properly, we can Improvise a cervical collar, NO immobilized by Complete, but it helps us to not move his neck.

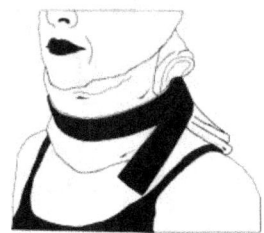

- The patient 's shirt or jacket can help us Immobilizing a senior member adosándolo his chest. Yes Same, a large handkerchief, can serve to make a sling. We can make it simple, it only supports the arm; or Compound, creating a reinforcement surrounding the trunk.

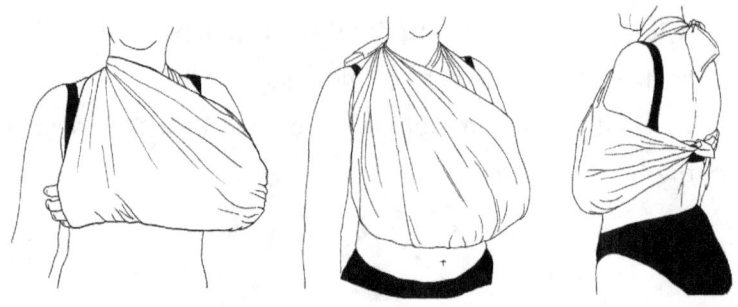

- A newspaper or magazine that involves a member, held with ribbons, you can serve to immobilize a doll or Any other member.

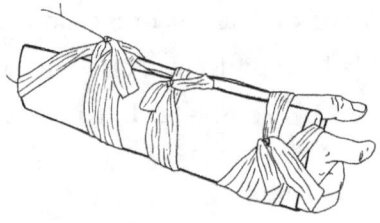

- For an elbow fracture can immobilize the member holding on to upper body.

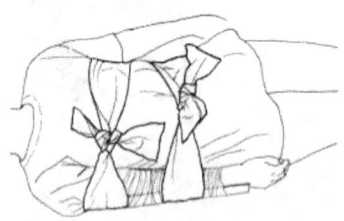

- A pillow or rolled blanket conveniently they can serve to immobilize an arm or a foot, placing around, and tying it with ribbons or bands.

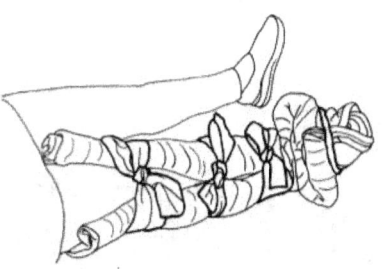

- To immobilize a joint or an open fracture, We can use two tablets, placed on either side of the Joint, joined by tape at its ends.

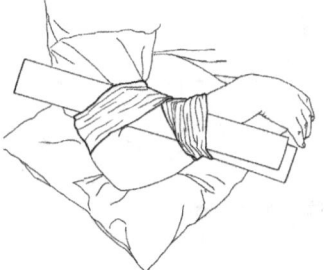 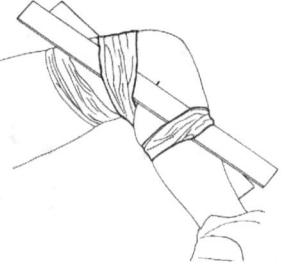

- If we freeze a lower limb, we can Do so using the healthy limb as tablet andtie them with Tapes passing through the hips, knees and ankles. We must Put a cushion (preferably rigid) between the two Legs.

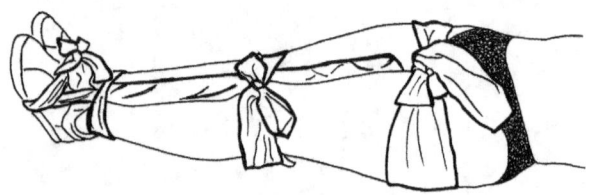

- We can use a long board or a broomstick I attached to the lower member and tied with ribbons or bands, which immobilize the area very well.

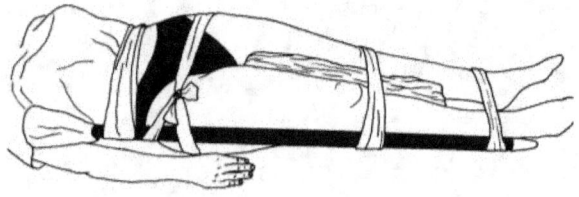

8. BITES AND SCRATCHES

Bites are very common, especially among children. Among these, those that cause skin breakdown, as all puncture wounds, they offer a high risk of infection and also present risk of injury to adjacent areas, such as tendons and Joints.

Human bites can be more dangerous than most animal bites, as there are microbes anaerobic in some human mouths that can cause difficult to treat infections. It is even possible that someone with an infected human bite, especially in hand, requires hospitalization for intravenous antibiotics.

What to do?

- Wash hands thoroughly with soap
- If the wound is not bleeding, we will wash the area with soap smooth and running water for 3 to 5 minutes and cover
- With a clean napkin. We will not use in any case water hydrogen or alcohol
- If the wound is bleeding profusely, should be monitored bleeding by applying direct pressure with a piece of cloth clean and dry or gauze until the bleeding ceases. He recommended to raise the affected area. Do not use hydrogen peroxide or alcohol
- Seek medical assistance if:
    - Have swelling or pain

    - The bite occurred near the eyes or involves the hands, fists or feet

    - The victim has immunodeficiency, as there increased risk of wound infection

9. WOUNDS AND CUTS

If the wound is bleeding severely, call 9-1-1

Minor cuts and puncture wounds can be treated at home, taking into account the following steps:

- Wash hands with soap to avoid infection
- Thoroughly wash the wound with water and mild soap
- Use direct pressure to stop bleeding
- If the possibility of the wound contamination or reopen by friction, should be covered (once He has stopped bleeding) with a bandage that will not stick to the wound
- If the wound has been puncture, search for objects within the Bruised but not fumbling. If we found some not recommended to withdraw, but go to the emergency room. Also, if you can not see anything inside the wound, but missing a fragment of the object that caused it , seek medical care
- The following types of wounds are more likely to Infected bites, punctures, crushing injuries, dirty wounds, wounds on the feet and wounds that are not timely treatment
- ALWAYS consult with your doctor to assess vaccination tetanus, especially if the wound has been an object metal

What not to do?

- DO NOT assume that a minor wound is clean because you can not see dirt or debris inside it. Should always wash
- DO NOT breathe or blow on an open wound
- DO NOT clean a major wound, especially after the bleeding is under control
- DO NOT remove a long or deeply object embedded, or probe or removing debris from a wound, but seek medical attention
- DO NOT push exposed body parts but cover them with clean material until help arrives

10. BITES

Insect bites can cause skin reaction Immediate. Bites from ants and stings bees, wasps and hornets are usually very painful. It's more Probably mosquito bites, fleas and mites cause Itching than pain.

In most cases, they can be easily treated at home; However, some people have severe allergic reactions. This is a life - threatening allergic reaction called

Anaphylaxis requires urgent medical attention. Reactions severe can affect the entire body and occur in a short space of time. If untreated, they can become deadly.

What to do?

- Remove the stinger if present scraping part back of a plastic card or some other object edge straight. Do not use tweezers, since these can break the Sting and increase the amount of poison released
- Thoroughly wash the affected area with soap and water
- Cover the bite site with ice, never directly, For about 10 minutes, remove for 10 minutes repeat the process. If there are no ice, water use Sour (9 parts water to 1 vinegar). Do not use in AMMONIA any case it can be toxic by inhalation
- If necessary, take an antihistamine or apply creams reduce itching. If you do not know the medical history victim is better to wait to be managed by a physician.
- Observe the wound for several days to ensure that no signs of infection (such as increasing redness, temperature increase of

the area, swelling or pain)

- If bitten by ticks, bathe them in oil, petrolatum or other oily cream and hold for 30 minutes as Usually shed

For emergencies, call 911 if you have:

- Difficulty breathing, shortness of breath or wheezing
- Swelling anywhere on the face
- Tightness in the throat
- Feeling weak
- Bluish discoloration

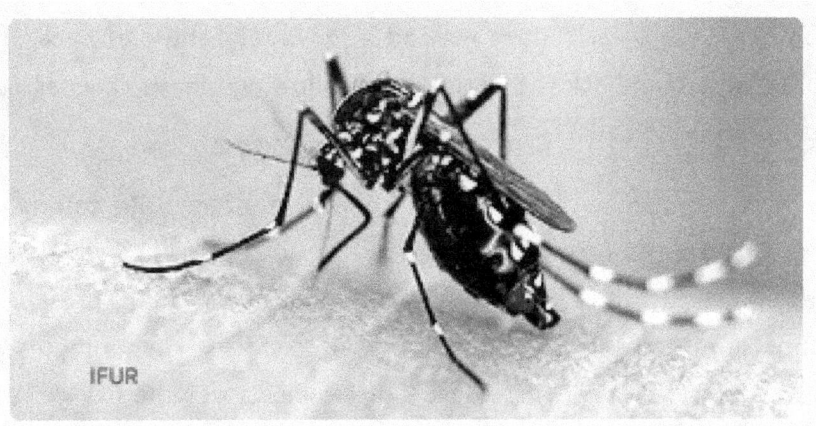

IFUR

11. NOSEBLEEDS

A nosebleed can be scary, but try keep calm. Most nosebleeds can be treated outside the hospital.

What to do?

If you start with a nosebleed, feel and tilt In front. Keep your head above your heart will make your nosebleeds less. Lean forward so that blood drain out of your nose instead of down and the part back of her throat. If you lean back the victim can swallowing blood. This can cause nausea, vomiting and diarrhea.

Use your thumb and forefinger to squeeze together the soft part of nose. This area is located between the tip of her nose and the edge hard, bony that forms the bridge of the nose. Keep doing pressure on the nose until the bleeding stops or for at least five or ten minutes. You can also place a cold compress or an ice pack over the bridge of the nose. Once he bleeding stops, do not do anything that could make again Start bleeding again, such as lean or blowing your nose.

12. CHOKING: OBSTRUCTION ROUTE AERIAL

If a person 's airway is blocked, you can Lose consciousness. To prevent this from happening, it is necessary that Learn some techniques.

Babies or children under one year

Place the baby face down, and back to you, She is holding her head and shoulders with his right arm. With The left hand to give five quick and pat dry between Shoulder blades. If that does not work, go back to baby face toward you and Lay it over his other arm. Place two fingers on the Lower half of the chest and apply pressure to five quick Below about 2 centimeters. At the same time, look inside Of the baby's mouth and place your finger on the tongue to view Obstruction.

Do not perform digital scans blindly. If there is not Baby response, activate the emergency system Continue to implement these techniques.

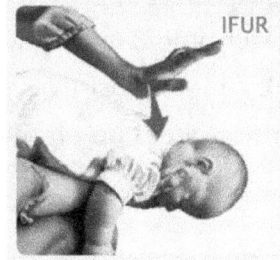 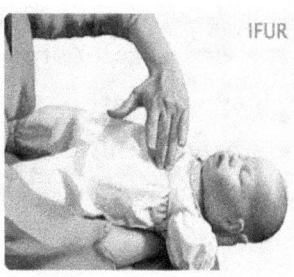

Children over one year

Pat on the back, and if conscious, have him cough, speak, or breathe. If you can not make any of the three, stand behind it and locate the lower tip of the sternum with his hand. Place the thumb and the rest of the hand into a fist this area and place the other hand over your fist.

Make Pressure in the stomach of the victim in upward direction Quick way. Push until you exit the object is Obstructing the airway.

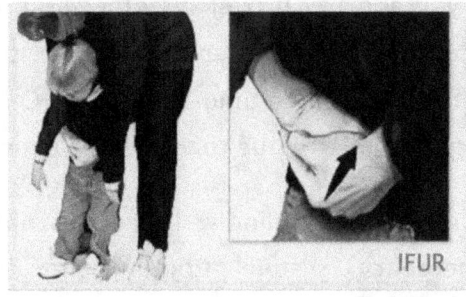

Adults

Stand behind the victim. Locate the lower tip of sternum with his hand. Place the thumb and the rest of the Hand into a fist over this area and place your other hand on his fist. Perform pressure on the stomach of the victim upward direction quickly. Push until you exit the object blocking the airway.

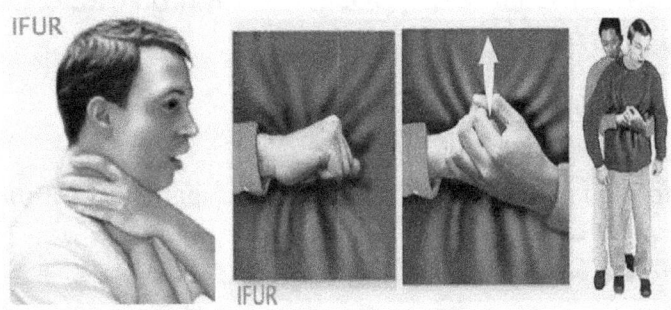

Auto - Heimlich

If we are alone in a choking situation, Can we realize the Heimlich maneuver ourselves.

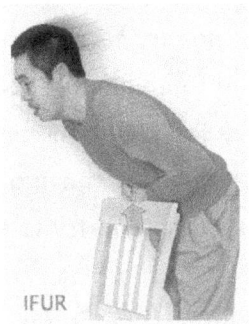

13. FOREIGN BODIES IN EYES, NOSE AND HEARD FOREIGN BODIES IN THE EYES

When a foreign body enters the eye, the patient Lagrimear starts flashing and unconsciously, to treat Ejecting out.

What to do?

- Prevent the victim rub the eye, not increase injury
- Wash your hands and try to locate the foreign body the lower eyelid gently lowering or raising the top We will ask you to look in all directions to inspect while the eye
- If it is embedded, not try to remove it , cover the eye with a Clean gauze and go to an emergency room
- If the foreign body is visible on the surface of the globe Eye and is not embedded, try moving it to the outside with a splash of water or saline and try to Remove it with the tip of a moistened gauze
- Seek medical attention if symptoms persist

FOREIGN BODY IN THE NOSE

The introduction of a foreign body in the nose is usually very common in children. You can become a serious problem if cause damage to the nasal cavity or if the foreign body penetrates airway.

What to do?

- Breathing through the mouth while the object is in the nose, as It can be introduced further
- Blowing gently mucus to try it Pull
- Unless the subject is very close to the entrance of the nose And clearly visible, there is little that can be done without help Professional, because if we introduce an object to remove it is Runs the risk of pushing the object into or Down
- Move the victim to an emergency room watching your Breathing

FOREIGN BODY IN THE EAR

Nor is it common to penetrate a foreign body in the ear. The most common are usually insects, which are housed usually in the outer ear. You may have impaired hearing and complain of strange sounds and even pain.

What to do?

- Do not try to remove it with any instrument except display In the vicinity of the pinna
- Tilt your head to the affected side and shake her with smoothness
- If it is an insect can be introduced warm water To leave outwardly
- We will move the victim to a health center as it runs danger of infection

14. CONVULSION

Seizures occur when the body of a person shakes rapidly and uncontrollably. During seizures, the muscles of the individual contract and relax as repetitive.

These seizures are caused by electrical activity disorganized and sudden in the brain. It can be disturbing witness the occurrence of seizures, but despite his appearance, most seizures are relatively harmless. They usually last from 30 seconds to 2 minutes; without But if a prolonged seizure occurs, or if present multiple crises on without the person he regains consciousness between them, is a situation medical emergency.

FEBRILE SEIZURES

About 3 to 5% of healthy children between 9 months to 5 years will have a seizure due to fever. Children small are most commonly affected. Most febrile seizures are triggered by a rapid temperature rise over 39 ˚C. The majority It occurs within the first 24 hours of a disease and not necessarily when the fever is at its highest point. From It is indeed not the speed of temperature elevation or the grade fever which seems to trigger seizures. To often the seizure is the first sign of fever.

What to do about a seizure?

- The main objective is to prevent the victim is injured, protecting it from a fall and from lying on the floor in a safe area. Must be removed furniture or other objects cutting nearby

- Place a cushion or pillow to rest your head boy
- Loosen tight clothing, especially those they are around the neck
- Place the victim in recovery position (PLS); whether presents vomiting, this helps ensure they are not sucked Into the lungs
- Stand beside the victim until he recovers or until
- You have professional medical assistance, which we will
- Previously warned
- If the child has fever at the time it occurs the seizure must focus our attention on lowering fever. We use physical means, for cloths place it on the forehead, English or underarms, or by entering the child in a bathtub with warm water, never cold. once it has stopped convulsing and only if the child is awake, administer the appropriate dose weight an antipyretic, provided the doctor has indicated previously

What not to do?

- Not restrict movement or move, unless it is In danger

- Do not insert any object between the teeth during a crisis convulsive, not our fingers

- Do not try to stop convulsing as it has no control on the crisis and it is not aware of what is happening

- We do not administer any medication orally to that the convulsions have stopped and the victim is fully awake and alert

15. ASTHMA ATTACKS

What is asthma and how is it treated?

Childhood asthma is an inflammatory disease of the airways which manifests in childhood with symptoms such as cough, either dry, persistent, at rest or with exercise; chest sounds, pain or chest tightness and shortness of breath.

The defining feature of asthma is inflammation of the bronchi, leading to become thicker and present less space for the passage of air, so will produce more mucus and will shrink more easily.

These symptoms can be triggered or worsened in the presence of allergens, drugs, climatic factors, stress, nervousness, among others. chronic disease that is manifested by exacerbations and requires ongoing treatment to control symptoms, prevent crises and reduce inflammation airways.

How to avoid the appearance of a flare Flare-ups occur

When any of the factors triggers causes inflammation of the airways and It limits the flow of air through them. It is appropriate to prevent this situation occurs, although asthma attacks unleashed By environmental factors it is difficult to avoid such exposure. Yes Were happening, is required to act immediately and that people who are in charge are familiar with the drugs commonly used by the child with the dose and the guidelines that will be followed in every situation.

If the crisis were to occur, the following act mode:

- Be sure not to leave it near the factor that triggered the crisis

- Be sure to use the drugs that have been ruled by the doctor for this situation, helping if necessary

- Provide a quiet environment and try to be relaxed

- Unzip the clothes you press the neck, chest or If desired waist and offer water to drink

- Help him to breathe during the crisis using methods diaphragmatic breathing

If despite implementing all these measures and after 15 minutes, the victim shows any of the following symptoms, ask for medical aid or transferred to an emergency room:

- If there is no improvement after 15 minutes

- If you're anxious and has difficulty speaking

- If you feel exhausted

- Lips and fingernails turn bluish

- The pulse exceeds 120 beats per minute

Common triggers of asthma attacks in the Medium:

· Allergens:

- Plant pollens, weeds or trees

- Dust mites and
- Epithelia of humans or animals

· Irritants unspecific:

- Snuff smoke or other fumes or vapors
- Indoors and charged environments
- Strong-smelling substances: sprays, cologne, alcohol, vinegar, varnishes, paints, etc.

· Climatic factors: fog, humidity, extreme cold or heat or sudden temperature changes

· Emotions: stress, anxiety, crying, laughing, nervousness

· Drugs: Drugs beta-adrenergic blockers

· Infections Respiratory: Colds from repetition, flu, sinusitis, etc.

· Physical exercise: it facilitates the entry of cold air to Lungs

· Other triggers:

- Disease (GERD)
- Food additives (sulfites, glutamate, tartrazine, etc.)
- Foods to which the child is susceptible or highly allergy
- Seeds, grains, flours

16. DIABETES MELLITUS

Diabetes is a chronic condition that occurs when the pancreas It is unable to produce enough insulin or when the body fails to use the insulin it produces. It is characterized by the presence of high concentrations of blood glucose. This circumstance alters the metabolism of carbohydrates, the Lipids and proteins.

Type 1 DM usually occurs in people under 30, and generally it termed as insulin-dependent diabetes.

Type 2 DM usually occurs in people older than 50 years.

Symptom

- Fatigue
- Disproportionate feeling of hunger or polyphagia
- Weightloss
- Excessive production of urine or polyuria
- Intense thirst or polydipsia

When symptoms are maintained over time uncorrected by providing insulin, you may see a box ketosis and coma, in which the patient has a serious life-threatening.

Treatment

Treatment consists of daily insulin delivery by Injections. Several types of insulin, to be described continuation:

- Ultrafast insulin action begins to take effect At 15 minutes after taken, acting more Intensity between 30 and 70 minutes.
- Acting insulin that begins to take effect 30 minutes after taken, acting with greater intensity between 1 and 3 hours after injection.
- SLOW INTERMEDIATE insulins or start action take effect 60 minutes after taken, acting with greater intensity between 3 and 6 hours after injection.

Dosages

The most common patterns of insulin are:
- Two, three or more doses, putting a mixture of insulin intermediate and fast, before breakfast, food, lunch or dinner

Insulin requirements will vary with age and under evolves his disease, so the disease forces periodic monitoring.

Physical exercise

Physical exercise improves glucose control and also decreases the amount of insulin. Patients with diabetes can and you should exercise daily. The most recommended is to low resistance or aerobic.

Before performing physical exercise should monitor blood sugar levels and take appropriate precautions; also you should carry carbohydrates of rapid absorption (glucose tablets, sugar cubes or fruit juices).

The extraordinary exercise, especially if it is severe, can cause severe hypoglycemia while it is performing and even 12 or 24 hours later, so glucose control is necessary strict and, if necessary, take extra meals to combat these hypoglycemia.

The performance of any physical activity is contraindicated if the

Patient is poorly controlled or has blood glucose levels high.

Excursions, trips, etc.

Whenever you go to make an exit, it is recommended that the patient carry:

- o Personal identification
- o Sugar and sugary drinks
- o Syringes and needles or injectors
- o Insulins necessary for the duration of the trip
- o Glucometer, lancets and test strips
- o Glucagon (in isothermal container, placed in a place Easily accessible). Indicated to hypoglycaemia
- o Treatment plan schedules and guidelines
- o Prepared food

Remember:

- If a diabetic person feel dizzy, shaking him Hands, speaking in a rare, see "fuzzy" has an attitude not habitual or cries for no reason, you may be suffering hypoglycemia
- If a diabetic person loses consciousness, possibly this I suffering from hypoglycemia, transfer to a center health or seek emergency medical care
- If you do not have a meter and we doubt if you file a hypoglycemia or hyperglycemia, act as if Try to hypoglycaemia ADMINISTERING SUGAR, as low blood glucose leads to increased RISK VITAL that an elevation of the same

MAIN ABBREVIATIONS

- DESA / DEA. Semiautomatic / Defibrillators
- DM. Mellitus diabetes
- FX. Fracture
- PCR. Cardiorespiratory arrest
- PLS. Lateral Security Position
- PR. Stop Breathing
- RCP. Cardiopulmonary resuscitation
- SVA. Advanced Life Support
- SVB. Basic Life Support
- TAC. Computed Tomography
- TCE. Traumatic brain injury
- TTO. Treatment
- TX. Trauma / Injury
- Oral vo

REFERENCE

1. Pérez Vigueras, J. Barrera Vallejo, AL. Adult and Pediatric Basic Life Support - CPR and management Semi-Automatic defibrillator – AED. Murcia. ED. IFUR 2015

2. Pérez Vigueras, J. Barrera Vallejo, AL. First Aid for teachers and parents. Murcia. Ed. IFUR 2015

3. 2015 AHA Guidelines for CPR and ECC

4. Pérez Alcaraz, J. Pérez Vigueras, J. Barrera Vallejo, AL. First Aid for First Responders. Murcia. Ed. IFUR 2015

5. Pérez Vigueras, J. Abrisqueta Garcia. J. Barrera Vallejo, AL Manual management, mobilization and transportation of victims. Murcia. Ed. IFUR 2015.

6. Pérez Vigueras, J. Barrera Vallejo, AL. My friend extinguisher. Murcia. Ed. IFUR 2015.

7. Neumar RW, Shuster M, Callaway CW, et. al. Part 1: executive summary, 2015 American Heart Association Guidelines Update for Cardiopulmonary Resuscitation and Emergency Cardiovascular Care. Circulation. 2015

8. Neumar RW, Shuster M, Callaway CW, et al. Part 1: executive summary: 2015 American Heart Association Guidelines Update for Cardiopulmonary Resuscitation and Emergency Cardiovascular Care. Circulation. 2015;132(18)(suppl 2). En prensa

9. Hazinski MF, Nolan JP, Aicken R, et al. Part 1: executive summary: 2015 International Consensus on Cardiopulmonary Resuscitation and Emergency Cardiovascular Care Science With Treatment Recommendations. Circulation. 2015;132(16)(suppl 1). in press

10. Nolan JP, Hazinski MF, Aicken R, et al. Part 1: executive summary: 2015 International Consensus on Cardiopulmonary Resuscitation and Emergency Cardiovascular Care Science With Treatment Recommendations. Resuscitation. In press

11. Institute of Medicine. Strategies to Improve Cardiac Arrest Survival: A Time to Act. Washington, DC: National Academies Press; 2015.

12. Pérez Vigueras J. Juárez Torralba J. et al. First involved in the emergency and hospital emergency. Advanced Life Support. Madrid. Aran editions, 2010.

13. Abrisqueta Garcia, J. Juarez Torralba J. Pérez Vigueras, J. Basic Manual management, mobilization and transportation of victims, injured and traumatized. Madrid. Aran editions, 2001.

14. Monteagudo Soto E., Pérez Vigueras, J. Evacuation and transfer of patients. Barcelona. Ed. Altamar, 2012.

15. Pérez Vigueras J. and others. Emergency Manual and Emergency Nursing. Murcia. Ed. Official College of Nursing of Murcia.

16. P. García Pradillo Pharmacology in nursing. Madrid. Ed. DAE, 2003.

17. Vigueras Pérez, J. Perea Lifante, Campillo FJ Pérez, JA Pérez Gracia, JM. I want to be a firefighter 2 - agenda of oppositions. Murcia. Ed. IFUR 2015

18. OPERATION WITH A SINGLE DUMP rescuer. Pérez Vigueras, J. Juarez Torralba, J. Abrisqueta Garcia. J. Rescue operation "turned a only rescuer "copyright© Murcia, 2006, RPI No. 08/2006/309

19. Pérez Vigueras, J. Perea Lifante, FJ. Campillo Pérez, J. I want to be firefighter - agenda of oppositions. Murcia. Ed. IFUR 2015.